Anna Mancini

# Tricks to Remember Your Dreams

*Why You Don't Remember Your Dreams And How To Dream Again*

Buenos Books America
www.buenosbooks.us

© Anna Mancini - www.amancini.com

ISBN: 978-1-963580-05-1

Imprint:
Buenos Books America LLC
www.buenosbooks.us

# INTRODUCTION

I spent almost all my life exploring the dream world and its connection to our waking life. When I started to teach my discoveries about dreams, I was surprised by the many people interested in this subject but telling me that they were unable to remember their dreams, or that they did not dream or had not dreamed for years, or that they could only remember a dream from time to time because it was a terrible nightmare. Of course, I decided to do something to help them open the doors of their inner world of dreams. That is why I wrote the present book, so that they too could enjoy all the benefits that normal dream activity can bring to their life.

Dreaming is far from being useless. We can do so many things in a dream state. For example, we can get news from a missing person or from a relative living in a remote place; we can communicate with a person in a coma or with a baby in her mother's womb; we can foresee our future; we can be warned of impending natural disasters or accidents; we can better manage our health; be guided in our career; or in our love life, and even locate lost items. All this is not hard to achieve, and you can even achieve much more with your dreams.

People who can remember their dreams well have a great advantage over others who don't because they have access to much more information that will help them improve their waking life and accelerate their personal growth. In this book, I will tell you how you can reactivate the ability to remember your dreams. I will speak about the different causes that usually block this ability and how to overcome these blocks in a natural way. In this book, you will find the solution to remembering your dreams by using the techniques that most appeal to you. Once the door of your dreams will be opened wide, you will be able to embark on an exciting journey into your inner world. You will better understand the functioning of your mind and body at the meeting point between your dreams and your reality. Through the exploration of your inner world, you will also discover the invisible world that permeates the tangible world but is not accessible to our senses. You will become aware of some aspects of your existence to which you had never before paid attention, but which could positively change your life. When you will have unlocked your ability to remember your dreams, you will have reached the first level of the art of dreaming.

Level "zero" is the one where you sleep normally but do not remember your dreams. The level below "zero" is where people suffer from insomnia. For them, I have written a book in which I share unusual information to help them find good sleep naturally and without drugs.[1] When you will be able to remember your dreams, you will have reached the first stage of the art of dreaming. Above this first level, there are higher and more interesting levels. According to the level reached, a person can travel in certain dream worlds; experience lucid dreaming; communicate clearly with other people (alive, dead, in their mother's womb or in a coma) and with animals and plants; visit other parts of the universe; be inspired to make inventions, literary or artistic works.

---

[1] Tricks to Sleep Better, Anna Mancini

# CHAPTER 1: The ABCs to remembering your dreams

When someone tells me he does not dream, at first, I ask him how many hours a night he sleeps, second, at what time he has his dinner and what he has for dinner and third, how he wakes up and what he does when he awakens. The answers to these three questions and the implementation of some very simple measures suffice most of the time to reactivate the dream capacity of most of the consultants. We all dream without exception because dreaming is a function absolutely necessary for the maintenance of life. This has been proved in scientific laboratories by the death of subjects deprived for a while from the REM phase of their sleep. So when people claim that they do not dream, it simply means that they forget their dreams. It would be easy for most of them to reactivate their ability to remember their dreams using the advice mentioned in this book.

## 1) It is important to sleep long enough to be able to remember your dreams well.

As a kid, I firmly believed that sleeping was useless, and I wanted to stop sleeping or drastically reduce my sleeping time, but fortunately, I never succeeded in this endeavor. Otherwise, I would never have learned that much about dreams and my life would have been dreams deprived like that of so many people who sleep too little to remember their dreams and who, therefore, cannot benefit from all the information that dreams convey to our "conscious mind" while we quietly sleep. It is possible to restore yourself physically with only around four hours of sleep and to behave almost normally at a physical level. However, in my opinion, this recharge is not enough to allow the optimal functioning of the brain that is required to be able to remember your dreams. According to experiments made in scientific laboratories, if you sleep only a few hours a night, you have only a short REM period. REM is the period in which a rapid movement of the eyes occurs, which is the period in which scientists believe we dream. According to them, it is only after eight hours of sleep that the REM periods become longer, up to an hour. Therefore, a long period of sleep puts us in much better conditions to dream more. I have not verified this scientific explanation since I do not have a laboratory at my disposal. However, from experience, I can say that a bad recharge of energy (due to insufficient sleeping time or to sleeping disorders) prevents or makes it extremely difficult to remember some dreams. The physical body can be regenerated after a few hours, but the energy recharge of the body is not optimal. We can compare this, for example, to the fact that, despite some difficulties and uneasiness, we are able to move, eat and live almost normally in our daily lives after a night without sleep. Our whole body moves almost normally, but our mind loses its sharpness and some of its usual capacities. We have memory gaps, it becomes harder to find the right words when we speak, we tend to be distracted and to provoke accidents, we make more mistakes, we are more easily stressed or afraid, and we are more likely to have negative emotions, we are prone to make bad decisions, we have difficulties concentrating our mind on intellectual tasks, sight, hearing and even taste decrease, etc.... I never met anyone sleeping only four hours a night who could tell me a dream. Naturally, there may be exceptions. The phenomenon of dreams and sleep is a vast realm, and a lot is yet to be discovered.

For the people who sleep too little, it is very easy to resume remembering their dreams. They just have to sleep longer, and they will almost always naturally remember some dreams. Sometimes, it is enough to sleep one or two hours more to reach this encouraging result. By extending their sleeping time, their energy recharge is improved, which makes it possible for their brain to be more performant and to recall some dreams.

Waking up instantly after a few hours of sleep with a brain as active as in the waking state and without the usual transition from dreaming to waking is "abnormal." I have often noticed this kind of awakening in people who sleep only a few hours a night. This situation is caused by an imbalance in the energy meridians (the energy channels of the body in Chinese medicine). Often, there is an "energy void in the spleen," which can be remedied thanks to a few sessions with a good acupuncturist. But this is a sleep disorder, a subject that I discuss in more detail in another book.[2] For now, just remember that to dream clearly and to remember your dreams, you need to sleep long enough.

---

[2] Tricks to Sleep Better, Anna Mancini

We should not accumulate fatigue resulting from nights that are too short or disturbed sleep because it is much harder to be happy and, of course, to remember our dreams if we are tired. There are times in our life where we cannot sleep enough. This is the case, for example, of parents of newborns babies. Fortunately, these impediments do not last forever and maintaining good sleep throughout our life should be a priority. The sleeping time necessary for a good recharge of energy varies from person to person and according to the seasons. It makes no sense to try to reduce your sleeping time to gain time since, without a good recharge, you will be much less effective and much more prone to mistakes and bad decisions that may ruin your day and waste a lot of your daytime. Being tired, you will also hardly be able to benefit from intuition and sudden inspirations that could facilitate your life.

Organize yourself so that you can sleep as much as you need and wake up in a good mood and without forcing yourself to leave your bed reluctantly. With a good night recharge, you will be much more efficient, and your day will be a thousand times more pleasant and joyful. The way you sleep and the time you spend sleeping largely determine the quality of your life. In addition to allowing you to dream clearly, excellent sleep brings health, longevity, calm, good mood, good look, beautiful skin, and many other gifts. Sleep is precious. It's a real treasure, and everything should be done to preserve it. If you are one of the people who sleep too little to remember your dreams, well, sleep longer. Be aware that shortening your sleep time to have more waking time is not a good idea, if for that little gain, you have to sacrifice "your dream life" and rely only on the limited abilities of your "conscious mind" to guide you through your existence. To reschedule your sleep habits, simply program yourself to sleep longer. How can you do it easily?

When you lie in your bed, at the moment you are about to fall asleep, think in a detached way (the way you daydream looking at the landscape when you travel by train) that you can sleep longer and you can even imagine the time you want to wake up. If done at the right moment, this simple technique will instruct your subconscious to reprogram your sleep patterns. For some people, it may work the first time. Others, however, must repeat it several times. This is a simple but efficient self-hypnosis technique that can be used for multiple purposes. You can change it to your taste, for example, by imagining waking up in the morning by looking at the alarm clock that marks an hour later than your usual time, or imagining waking up in good shape and happy to get out of your bed. Elaborate your thought content in this regard, but always implement the technique at the right time. That is the exact moment when you are falling into sleep. You may alternatively visit an acupuncturist or a hypnotist. Consulting a chiropractor to check that everything is in place in your spine can also be greatly useful. The misalignment of the cervical vertebrae, particularly the first one, can significantly influence the quantity and quality of your sleep.

Needing only a few hours of sleep a night is often considered an advantage in our Western society that gives so little importance to true vitality and does not take into account the energy of the human body. Sometimes, some people, just by realizing that it is not actually advantageous for them to live without dreaming, change their sleeping habits without needing to use any reprogramming technique.

To conclude on this topic, I also absolutely do not recommend taking sleeping pills to sleep more. In addition to their side effects, they have a disastrous effect on the ability to dream. Instead, it is better to use some relaxing herbal teas such as lavender, chamomile, valerian, etc.

A lack of good sleep is indeed the most common cause why people do not remember their dreams, but there are also people who sleep long enough and who do not remember or remember very little about their dreams. In such a case, I ask these people:

## 2) At what time do you have your dinner? What do you usually eat for dinner? And how long after your dinner do you go to sleep?

Modern life means that many people who work far from home do not have the time or the means to have a good lunch. As a result, being very hungry in the evening when they come back home after a long day out, they tend to eat too much at dinner because it is their main meal. It is nice to have a generous dinner every now and then with family or friends, but having it every evening is not at all recommended for many reasons. Eating a lot in the evening just before going to sleep is bad for your health, weight, dreams, life, and energy recharge. Popular wisdom recommends eating like a king in the morning, like a prince at noon, and like a poor man in the evening.

Dinner should be very light. If it is not possible, you should have dinner at least four or five hours before going to bed. The ideal would be to eat enough at lunch so that you can almost completely skip dinner. If you are not in the process of digestion at night, your sleep will be more restorative, and it will be much easier to remember some dreams. Instead, people who have the habit of dining copiously and then falling asleep immediately in front of the television or after reading a few pages or even a few lines of a book, wake up most of the time without remembering a dream. Unfortunately, when they can remember a dream, it is only a nightmare caused by poor digestion. So, if you do not dream because of your dinners, it will be very simple to reactivate your dream skills. All you will have to do is gradually change your meal times and the consistency of your dinner. It would be better to organize yourself to eat enough for breakfast and lunch so that you will not be very hungry at dinner. If you can do it, try to skip dinner; you will immediately notice the difference in the quantity and clarity of your dreams. It will also allow you to sleep better and avoid most of the digestive nightmares.

Sometimes, when dining copiously is a lifelong habit, people have a big belly full of gas and stagnant stool; a belly in this state is a big obstacle for dreaming normally because it disturbs the circulation of the blood and causes nightmares due to the suffering of the physical body. I advise you to read the booklet by Laure Goldbright: *Colon Cleansing and its Benefits for Health and Skin*. In this book, you will find all the information necessary to solve this problem. I would like to add that it is important to provide a substantial budget to buy quality food, the most natural and the most alive food you can find on the market. If you only eat dead, fat, canned, frozen food, full of pesticides, and as cheap as possible, you will, of course, survive eating this way because the human body is incredibly resistant, but you won't have enough vitality to activate your brain properly and to be fully conscious both in your dreams and in your reality. Many people are not aware that, for example, feeling lonely, having cravings for sweets, or for addictive substances like tea, coffee or alcohol are often triggered by a lack of life energy in the body, mainly caused by "poor" food and fatigue due to bad sleeping habits. Saving money on food, just like saving time on sleeping, is not really a good idea. These are two extremely unfortunate choices that "reduce the standard of living," the "lifespan," and make it very difficult "to have a dream life." The good news is that it is never too late to change for better habits in these two areas of our life.

At this point, we have seen that by sleeping longer or changing the time of the dinner and/or its composition, the ability to remember their dreams is quickly restored in the majority of people. Waking up remembering some dreams is also a sign that you have had good sleep and that you are in good health. However, there are also cases in which a great abundance of a certain type of dream is the sign of an energy imbalance, an excess of sleep, or in some cases, poorly working bowels. When a person tells me that she sleeps long enough and goes to bed with a light stomach but does not remember her dreams and I observe that she does not have a swollen stomach, I ask this third question.

### 3) How do you generally wake up?

We do not have only one brain, the one in our head. Modern science has discovered that we have another one in the belly supposed to have two hundred million neurons and interact with what we consider our most important brain, that of the head. With a little self-observation, you will easily notice that when you wake up in the morning, the energy of the dreams is not yet totally in your head but in your belly and throughout your body. The brain in the head, just like the whole body, gradually wakes up, and none of them should be rushed. When you wake up, normally, the first brain (in the head) is not active. In other words, it is not emissive. It is in a state of receptivity, a receptivity that makes remembering your dreams easy. Once the brain becomes emissive, it is much harder to remember your dreams. The brain becomes emissive when we project ourselves into real life, for example, by thinking about our business, talking to someone or listening to news on the radio or television. To remember your dreams effectively, you should wake up slowly, sit calmly in your bed and you will sense the energy and the images and other contents of your dreams gradually reach your conscious mind. In this phase, it is advisable to stay in a relaxed, receptive and meditative state that is akin to the numbness that precedes your falling asleep. This relaxed and receptive state acts as a bridge that your dreams can use to reach your conscious mind. Many people who are used to remembering their dreams do so naturally without analyzing what happens when they remember their dreams. Of course, if you wake up stressed by the alarm of your clock or in the mental agitation caused by thinking about your worries, there will be little or no hope that you will remember your dreams effectively. In the best case, you will only remember some fragments of dreams or some nightmares. Even in these unfavorable circumstances, there may be some exceptions, especially when your "subconscious mind" strongly wants to communicate an important message to you. A quick and agitated awakening, in addition to making you forget your dreams, is detrimental to your brain and to your whole body. If you need to use an alarm clock, arrange to go to sleep so that you can wake up naturally a few minutes before the time the alarm rings. These few minutes will be precious for remembering your dreams. At the same time, they will be a blessing for the good health of your brain and for your nervous balance. If you wake up and begin your day calmly and peacefully, you will be more relaxed and efficient during the whole day.

To remember some dreams, it has been advised to wake up during a REM phase with the help of an alarm clock. This is a method that I do not recommend, on one hand, because it can create sleep disorders; on the other hand, because it is possible to remember your dreams naturally without stressing your body. It is important to respect our body and its sleep cycles. The better the body is treated, the more it will cooperate to help you in the art of dreaming.

As you have understood, dreaming is not just a mental process; it involves the whole person who dreams, mind and body. And the body plays an important role in the dream process.

**Your body is indeed a bridge between the visible world and the invisible world that surrounds you.**

I would like to add that computers, tablets and phones should always be turned off when you sleep and when you wake up. You may use them only after you have written down your dreams. At this moment, they may trigger the recall of more dreams. When I check my mail after writing down my dreams, I often notice that some of the dreams I have just noted were premonitory dreams containing the information emailed to me. It is as if I had received the email first in my dreams and then in my reality. Reading my emails also regularly triggers in my mind the recall of some more dreams. I have also tried a technique to remember dreams better that is often mentioned in the literature about dreams. It consists of staying in bed and lying on one side and then on the other side. This is less effective than sitting in my bed, and moreover, with this technique, I greatly risk falling back asleep for a new sleep cycle and waking up tired from too much sleep. Sleeping too much is as bad for health as not sleeping enough.

For now, we have seen that to be able to remember your dreams, you need to get enough sleep, have a light dinner or dine long before you go to sleep, and finally wake up slowly and quietly. If you do all this but still cannot remember your dreams, then try the following boosts.

# CHAPTER 2: Boosts to better remember your dreams

We do not always dream with the same intensity, with the same clarity and in the same way. It even happens that "strong dreamers" wake up sometimes without remembering any dreams. This is so strange for them to have forgotten all what they "did" during all these hours spent in bed that they often use techniques to grasp, nevertheless, some snippets of their dreams. You can also use the following techniques that I have listed under the "self boosts" category because they do not require external help. You can do it on your own.

<u>1) Boost to grasp some dreams, images or snippets of your dreams</u>

You have woken up slowly and silently after a good night's sleep, and yet you do not remember any dream. Do not be discouraged. Try the following:

## a) Feel the gradual awakening of your body

Notice the state of mind in which you have awakened, let your emotions flow into your conscious mind. If you cannot remember your dreams as soon as you wake up, get in touch with your body. This will bring back some memories, images, emotions or snippets of dreams. Try to feel each part of your body and to feel its gradual awakening. Also, observe your mood. How do you feel? Are you happy to start a new day? Are you in a bad mood? Or do you feel tired and depressed, with no enthusiasm for your life? Even when they seem unpleasant, let these feelings and emotions come to your conscious mind and observe them without judgment. Take note of your state in your notebook. When you do so, take your time, form all the letters slowly and calmly. As you write in such a relaxed way, other fragments of dreams and often whole, clear and precise dreams that you will be surprised to have forgotten, will come back to your mind.

## b) Do not be discouraged

If after having done that, you do not get any results, again do not be discouraged. Rather, write in your notebook what you did the day before. To do so, try to remember your previous day starting from the evening and ending in the morning. You can also do this exercise the night before going to sleep; this will be a workout to improve your memory in general. If you do this exercise in the morning, fragments of dreams, information, insights and emotions will appear in your mind. Since the dreamer is the same person as the one who lives his reality, his dreams and reality are connected, i.e. there is continuity between the dreams and the reality of the same person. Unfortunately, many people in the Western world are not sufficiently enough recharged energetically to be able to fully feel this continuum of human life from dream to reality and vice versa and to learn how to make better use of it. After having noted your reality of the day before, walk a little in your room, open the windows and breathe. Start your new day with the determination to be aware and conscious of what you will experience this day. This means that you will do many things consciously instead of doing them automatically. This way, you will see that always "acting consciously" is not that easy. We often have gotten into the habit of living in a distracted way, without paying attention to what we are doing, without looking at the people we meet, without listening to the noises from our environment, and without paying attention to odors. Cultivating the fact of acting consciously instead of automatically during your waking life will help you develop a kind of "consciousness" in the dream state that will help you remember your dreams.

Take note: Training yourself to do every action with all your consciousness (instead of doing them automatically) when you are awake will greatly improve the recall of your dreams.

### c) **Perform some creative activities**

Upon awakening, you can do some creative, relaxing activities. This is also a great way for those who cannot remember their dreams to recover some snippets of their dreams or some dreams fully, some impressions, images, or intuitions. These same creative activities carried out during the day can also produce the same results. The type of creative activity does not matter. What is important is to do it in a relaxed way, having fun like a child. Here are some examples of creative activities that work well: invent a story, draw or scribble, randomly arrange small pebbles of different colors and shapes, choose cards from a bunch and place them in front of you as you like, or put objects or small stones in places of your home where you are attracted to do so at this moment. If you like reading and if you have a library, choose a book. Open it randomly with your eyes closed, place your index finger somewhere on a page, then open your eyes and read what is under your finger. By doing so, we often pick up something related to our dreams, and this has the effect of making them come back to our mind. Try and see what works best for you. Creative or playful activities put us very easily in contact with our subconscious mind and bring out images, emotions, snippets of dreams, and sometimes even clear and precise entire dreams.

### d) **Think about your projects and the people you know**

If the techniques mentioned above did not work for you, try this. Review in your mind, in a receptive, calm and relaxed way (as when you are on a train looking at the landscape) the faces of the people you know. Think in the same way about your activities, your projects, etc. This can trigger the recall of certain dreams for the good reason that, as I said above, dreams and reality are connected and because your "subconscious mind" constantly creates your waking life and projects you into your future. It often happens that during the day, an activity, a gesture, a meeting, a poster, a phone call, an odor brings back to the mind a clear and precise dream of which, however, in the morning, there seemed to be not the slightest trace. The strange impressions of *déjà vu* stem from the fact that we have already seen some places or experienced some situations in our dreams, but that upon awakening, we have forgotten part of or all our dreams. If you effectively observe the links between your dreams and your reality over a long period, you will be able to see that everything we experience in waking life has been first programmed by the "subconscious mind." The events taking place in your reality are first programmed into your dream energy, generally overnight for the next day, but also sometimes some days, weeks or years before. In reality, everything happens as if we were living our lives upside down. It is not the conscious mind that drives the boat of our existence, but our subconscious forces, like it or not. We should rather be in tune with our subconscious forces to live a more harmonious and enjoyable life. This tuning also allows us to avoid some wrong choices made by our limited rational mind. Paying attention to your dreams every morning, you will gradually become more in tune with your "subconscious mind" (soul, higher self, call it what you prefer) and communicate better with it.

However, our ego and our rational mind are also involved in the art of dreaming, and they are important too. We just need to learn how to use them better and get them to cooperate with our "subconscious mind."

To remember your dreams well, your brain must also get enough exercise when you are awake.

### e) **Train your brain during the day so that it will be in shape to remember your dreams**

If you do not make your brain work enough while you are awake, it will also tend to be lazy while you sleep. If you have problems remembering your dreams, make your brain work a little more during the day, especially in the evening before going to sleep. To do this, you can write something, solve problems, invent solutions, and imagine alternative conclusions to a story. During the day (but not at night, as this can cause insomnia), read funny stories and laugh. If you have been out of school for a long time, go back to learning something, such as a foreign language or start an artistic activity. We should continue to learn throughout our lives to keep our brain active, dynamic and alive. Otherwise, the brain becomes lazy, the same way our body becomes lazy when we do not move enough. Even the eyes become lazy in their own way. One of the consequences of this is the spasm of the eye muscles that, through a towing effect, spreads throughout the body. For this reason, eye relaxation techniques are very useful not only to improve vision but also to help remember our dreams better.

**f) Using eye relaxation techniques to dream better**

The eyes play an important role in the dream process and in access to the subconscious. Science does not know exactly why, but in scientific laboratories, it has been discovered that the eyes move very quickly during the REM phase of sleep. REM means rapid eye movement. I do not have a laboratory to check this fact, but one day I saw a dog sleeping with his eyes wide open while it was in a REM phase, and I could observe this phenomenon that seemed really strange to me because the dog's usual gaze had disappeared. For a while, I have practiced techniques of relaxation of the eyes to improve my vision. This is how I could observe the positive effects of these techniques on the quality of sleep and the recall of dreams. This is simply because when the eyes are relaxed, the whole body tends to follow this trend, and we sleep better if we go to bed in a relaxed state. When we are relaxed, we dream better, and we also have more opportunities to remember our dreams. Here are three simple yet highly effective eye relaxation techniques. You can use them in the evening just before going to bed and complete them with the self-hypnosis technique I mentioned earlier that must be done when you are about to fall asleep. You can also practice them during the day. These three eye relaxation techniques are:

- looking at all the details of an image,

- palming,

- swinging to the right and to the left.

I invite you to read an interesting book on eyesight written by Dr. William H. Bates (1860-1931), a New York ophthalmologist, and entitled: *A perfect view without glasses, the cure of imperfections*. There are many editions of this book; many of them have been abbreviated. I advise you to consult a full version (about 400 pages) because in those that have fewer than 200 pages, unfortunately, the essential is missing.

<u>Look at the details of an image:</u>

This is very easy to do. Take a picture or image that you like and that contains many details. For example, I sometimes do this exercise myself to relax during the day, with a picture representing three dolphins jumping out of the water and that I bought during one of my vacation in Crete. It reminds me of the holidays and of the nice person who painted it. I quietly observe a very small part of the painting, for example, every tooth of the dolphin with an open mouth. My gaze passes quietly on every detail of the painting. I do this by hiding my right or left eye with my hand, and then I do the same with the other eye. After, I repeat the exercise with both eyes. This triggers the relaxation of my eyes and consequently helps the relaxation of my whole body.

Palming: Palming is an eye relaxation exercise that is very effective for also relaxing the whole body. To do this, wash your hands. Rub them to feel some heat coming into your palms, then cross them and cover your eyes with your hands without pressing on your eyeballs, but to hide the light. Once you have placed your hands, relax and imagine a black object, the blackest possible or a black dot, in the most passive and relaxed way. Do this exercise in the evening before going to sleep and complete it with the self-hypnosis technique explained above to suggest to yourself that you will remember your dreams. You can do this with another color; it works the same because focusing the mind on something brings relaxation.

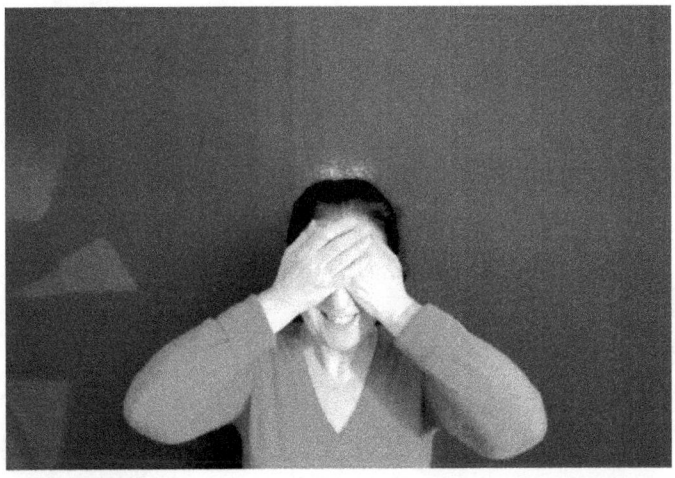

Swinging: The oscillations of the body on the right and on the left allowing the eyes to move naturally due to movement and without effort will relax your eyes and, at the same time, all your body. Complete this exercise with the self-hypnosis technique explained above, just before falling asleep. Avoid doing it right before you go to sleep, it is best to do it during the day.

In general, all the exercises you can do to relax your eyes will also have the effect of relaxing the whole body and improving your sleep and therefore the recall of your dreams. Of course, this will also improve your eyesight, and many people have gotten rid of their glasses by applying Dr. Bates' methods.

At this point, if you still cannot remember your dreams, try the following boosts.

<u>2) Material boosts to remember your dreams:</u>

**a) The effects of quartz on dreams**

At a time in my life, while I had already done a lot of personal work on dreams, I started to have many dreams in which I saw some crystals, in particular, quartzes and very beautiful gems. These dreams were so pleasant that they made me want to go to stores where they sell minerals. I was in Paris, where there are several good stores selling stones. I bought some stones and a few books on their properties, and then I had the idea to check in my dreams what I had read about the stones. To do so, it was enough for me to put them (one at a time) under my pillow and to sleep normally. In the dream state, my perceptions are much more extensive than when I am awake, and I can feel the effects of the stones on my body and on my mind. You can also learn to do the same. It's not difficult. I could sense the influence of some stones on my body and mind in my dreams, and sometimes, it was consistent with what I had read in the books, sometimes not. Some other stones provoked no effect in my dreams and in my reality. Among all the stones that I have tried, the clear quartz had the most spectacular and interesting effect on the art of dreaming. Indeed, I could observe that this quartz is an amplifier of thought and the recall of dreams. It makes it possible to dream more, to have clearer dreams and to remember them much easier. You can also experiment for yourself on the properties of quartz. For this, go to a shop of minerals and choose a nice quartz tip as clear as possible. Choose with your intuition the crystal that most attracts you. Before using it, pass it under water to clean it from all the influences it has accumulated before reaching you. Objects and places absorb thoughts, emotions, and energy. After doing this, place your crystal under your pillow and sleep normally. You will test the effectiveness of quartz, but for that, you need to find the crystal that's right for you. Its size is not what matters most. Here is a photograph of very effective quartz that I have been using for years and that I bought on the banks of the Hudson River in New York City.

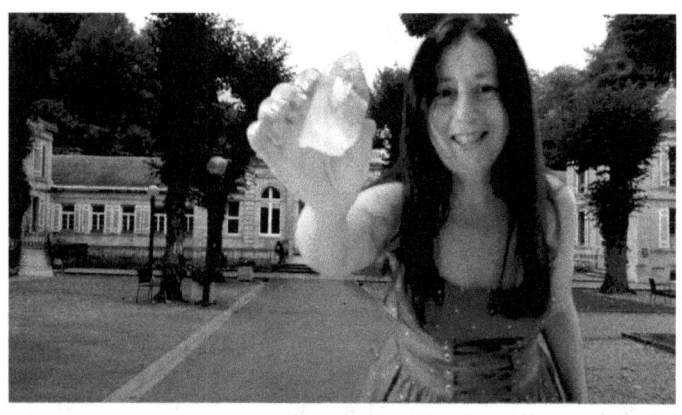

I had bought a much larger one in Paris, thinking it would be even more effective, but it is not as effective as the one I bought in New York. Here is a photograph of my quartz acquired in Paris. Next to it, there is a statuette that is a reproduction of an original rediscovered by archaeologists in the remains of the temples of Malta. These temples were built more than 6000 years ago, and it is thought that these statuettes of sleeping women refer to the spiritual practice of the art of dreaming. If I could go to sleep in one of these temples or put a recently discovered artifact under my pillow, I could learn more.

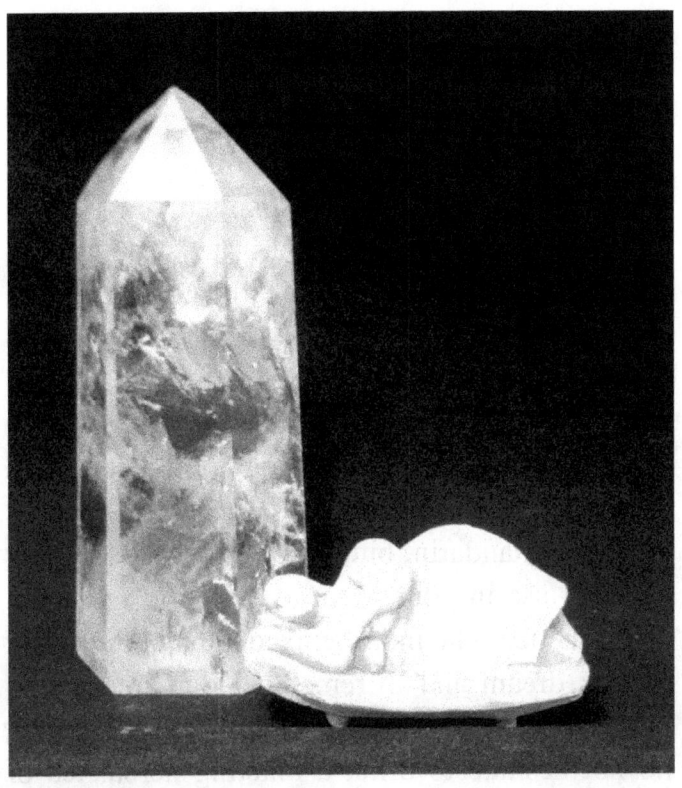

You can also place quartz in a glass bottle filled with water that you will leave for a few hours in the sun. Just drink some of this water before going to sleep. You will notice that your dreams are much brighter and that it is much easier for you to remember them. Naturally, you must be honest and consistent with yourself. If you go to bed immediately after eating like a pig, do not hope that the crystal, alone, as if by magic, will allow you to have clear dreams. This also applies to the other means that I will now present.

**b) Clary sage essential oil:**

A few drops of clary sage essential oil on a cotton pad placed in a cup of warm water near the bed will help you remember your dreams. (You can also use an effuser). Clary sage has a slightly hypnotic effect. It should not be used if you are stressed because, in this case, it could cause insomnia. Don't use it if you do not like its smell. There are other relaxing essential oils, such as lavender, mandarin, bitter orange or jasmine, that you can use in your room to help you relax and dream better. The more relaxed we are, the easier it is to dream and to remember our dreams. To increase your level of relaxation, in the evening, do not hesitate to drink a relaxing herbal tea of your choice (in small quantities to avoid having to get up to go to the bathroom during the night). Choose the best quality of herbal tea you can find, organic and loose, instead of bags. I particularly appreciate lavender tea that helps me have a deep and peaceful sleep. Of course, use the purest water possible to make herbal tea, one with very few minerals. You can also distill tap water to easily obtain very pure water. Type "water distiller" in a search engine to obtain information on water distillation and distillers available on the market.

When I am stressed, I take some magnesium because stress provokes magnesium deficiency, and so it is a vicious circle. I discovered a source of magnesium that outperforms everything that exists on the market called "oil of magnesium."

## c) Oil of magnesium is an excellent source of magnesium:

I found this product doing research on the Internet. One day, I was very stressed when I returned from a trip that had gone wrong, and I had the idea of typing on Google: "What minerals do we lose when we are stressed?" From one thing to another, I came to a site that sold this "magnesium oil." When I read the articles that advertised the many advantages of this product, it seemed too good to be true, and I thought it was a scam. However, my intuition told me to try it, and I listened to it as usual. This product was not expensive, and trying it did not involve big risks. Finally, I found the product in a store near my home, but you can also easily buy it online. "Magnesium oil" is a natural remedy that effectively helps with the magnesium deficiency that we all suffer when we are in a state of stress. "Magnesium oil" is actually not oil but a slightly viscous translucent liquid. It is seawater mixed with mineral water. It comes from a fossil sea discovered a few years ago in the Netherlands. This seawater contains natural magnesium of excellent quality. Just put a little bit on your skin every day and you will feel the benefits very quickly. The skin absorbs magnesium much better than the digestive system. For my part, before knowing the "magnesium oil" that I now use regularly, I was not able to take magnesium without my digestive system being completely disturbed. The only magnesium I could bear was the homeopathic one. Magnesium oil is an excellent product that I strongly recommend. It helps relax and relieves muscle pain and tendinitis due to stress. Stress is one of the greatest enemies of sleep and dreams. Fortunately, there are many ways at our disposal to help us relax: yoga, acupuncture, meditation, walks in nature, sports, reading, or the eye relaxation techniques mentioned above. Choose what is most effective for you. Making a habit of quietly writing down your dreams or feelings in case you don't yet remember your dreams in the morning will also help you be much more relaxed throughout the day. Try to go to sleep already relaxed and just before falling asleep you can decide that you will sleep very well, that you will dream well and remember your dreams. You can use the well-known technique of a glass of water. To do this, just fill a glass of water, drink half of it and then leave it on your night table; the next morning, when you drink the other half, you will remember your dreams. This is an example of self-suggestion; it is up to you to imagine the self-suggestion that will be more effective for your mind. If all that has been mentioned above has not worked for you yet, then it is time to ask for help from your loved ones and to try one of the "external boosters."

### 3) External dream recall boosters

The American people were lucky to have had Edgar Cayce among them, who lived from 1877 to 1945. When Edgar Cayce was in a self-induced hypnotic trance, he was able to do incredible things and, above all, to train people in the art of dreaming. He was also able to remember parts of dreams that the consultants themselves had forgotten. This was an extraordinary and very useful talent. Unfortunately, Edgar Cayce is no longer alive and cannot help you! In France, as far as I know, we did not have a character like Edgar Cayce. However, in the nineteenth century lived a man who was very interested in lucid dreams. His name was Hervey de Saint Denys. He was very creative regarding the experiments he did in the dream state. Hervey de Saint Denys describes in his book, *Dreams and How to Guide Them*, how he had managed to help a friend, who told him that he never dreamed, to remember a dream of the first sleep.

## a) **Hervey de Saint Denys' trick to help a friend remember a dream**

Hervey of Saint Denys (1822-1892), who wrote in 1867 his famous book about lucid dreaming, was a sinologist, professor at the College de France and member of the French *Academie des Inscriptions et belles lettres*. He had lucid dreams from childhood. And he kept a diary of his dreams starting from the age of fourteen. In his book that became the bible of lucid dreaming in the West, he describes the many experiments he did on dreaming. A lucid dream is a dream in which one is aware of dreaming and in which one has the possibility to decide to change the course of the dream, or to do whatever one decides, like flying or jumping from a cliff, or even eating a lot of chocolate. Here is an excerpt from the book by Hervey de Saint Denys that I have translated from the French version, to help you discover the trick he had imagined to help a friend remember a dream. You, too, can use this technique asking someone to help you.

> *A close friend, with whom I took a long trip and who was interested in my research, strongly pretended that he had never had a dream in its first sleep. I had woken him many times a short time after he had fallen asleep, and he had always assured me in good faith that he could not remember any dream. One evening while he had been sleeping for about half an hour, I approached his bed. I said in a low voice some military commands: Present arm! Shoulder arm! etc., then, I woke him gently.*
>
> *-Well, I said, this time did you dream of anything?*

*-Nothing, absolutely nothing, as far as I know!*

*-Search well in your mind.*

*-I'm searching, and there I find only a very complete period of mind annihilation.*

*-Are you sure?*

I asked then: "*Did you see a soldier?*" At the word, "*soldier,*" he was as if struck by a sudden reminiscence, "*It's true!*" He told me, "*Yes, now I remember. I dreamed that I saw a military parade. But how did you guess that?*"

I asked him permission to keep my secret until I had repeated the experiment. This time I murmured to him the terms inherent in the horsemanship, and, as soon as he was awake, an almost identical conversation took place between us. At first, he had no dream at all in mind, then he remembered, according to my indications, what my words had triggered, and, put in this way of reminiscences, he also recovered the memory of several previous visions, of which my intervention had disturbed the course. Shortly after this second experiment, I made a third one that was no less successful. Instead of using the word as a means of influencing the dream of my travel companion, I used small bells that I gently shook....

If you are not willing to use Hervey de Saint Denys' trick or cannot get someone to help you in doing so, then why not try the possibility of discreetly using the effect of the brain waves of other dreamers to help you remember your dreams?

**b) Taking benefit of the brain waves of other dreamers to help you recall your own dreams:**

One summer day, while I was writing in my room under the roof in Paris, my neighbor's cat named Mistigri came in for a visit entering by the window, which she did very often because she liked the atmosphere that emanates from the fact of writing and she also enjoyed drinking the water that I used to put in a bowl near the window to humidify the room where I worked. That's how my place became the neighborhood cats' best bar. That day, after drinking a little water, instead of returning to the rooftops of Paris, Mistigri went on my bed and fell asleep. I was awake and at work, and I appreciated her relaxing presence while she rested in peace far from her kittens. After ten minutes, however, her four kittens came in by the window, drank some water and went to sleep next to their mother. I found myself with five cats sleeping in my room, which triggered in me the desire to sleep too. It was too difficult to resist their powerful brain and body waves. I laid down beside the cats and immediately fell asleep too. When I woke up, they were all gone. This fortuitous experience gave me the idea of testing the effect of other people's brainwaves on dreams and sleep. For doing so, I asked some friends and relatives if they could sleep in the same room for at least one night. I started with one person at a time to test what the effect of a certain person's presence was on my dreams, my sleep and my energy field. Then, I had the idea to test the effect of a large group of people on my sleep, dreams, and energy level. Since my Paris apartment was not spacious enough to sleep in the same room with, let say, fifty people, I took a youth hostel card and went to sleep in crowded dormitories. This way, I could observe the effect on my dreams and my reality of the brainwaves of a group of sleeping people. I do not enter into detail. I want to come to what interests us most: dream recall.

When you sleep in a place where many other people are sleeping, you benefit from the group pulling effect. This balances your body's energy and, among many other benefits, gives you a boost to get back to better sleeping patterns and remember your dreams. Of course, you need to be equipped with earplugs and an eye mask if you are sensitive to noise and light. If you are unable to sleep during your first night in a dormitory, you will certainly sleep the next night because you will be tired and because of the group effect. Therefore, book for at least two nights to enjoy the special effect of the brainwaves of a group of sleepers. I do not know if there are scientific laboratories where they study and measure the energy exchanges between the brains and the bodies of sleeping people, but I know from experience that brains and bodies exchange information and energy both in the waking state and in the dream state. This phenomenon has also been observed by other people who have carefully studied their dreams.

Furthermore, it is not necessary to have a scientific laboratory to test the effect of a group on your sleep and on your dreams; just go to sleep in a big dormitory and check for yourself. The intense exchange of energy and information exchange that occurs between sleeping people is a vast field of research. You can take advantage of this phenomenon to help you reactivate the memory of your dreams and restore the natural rhythms of your body and improve your sleep patterns. This can be of great help in case of jet lag because you will benefit from the energy of the group that will help you immediately put your body in harmony with the natural energies of the place. If you do not like sleeping next to strangers, try this alternative: Go to sleep at your mother's house. If your mother has good sleeping/waking rhythms, this is a great chance for you because she will be of incredible help to help you recover quickly from jet lag. In such a case, do not take melatonin or some other remedy. Instead, try this: Go to sleep at her house. It will be much more effective. Since our mother's body made ours, our body tunes itself very quickly with our mother's sleeping/waking rhythms. If your mother has a habit of dreaming well and remembering her dreams, this will also help you remember your dreams. It's very powerful, but if you cannot do it for one reason or another, you can try doing the same with a member of your family. It may also work, but it is, of course, less efficient. As you can see, many interesting and useful experiences on dreaming and sleeping can be done using only your daily life as a laboratory.

If you do not want to go to sleep next to other people and you want to stay at home, you can also benefit from the help of other people by doing the following, although it may be much less effective.

## c) Use the dragging effect of objects belonging to people who dream well.

During my observations on dreams, I could observe that the information of the objects that I placed beside the bed or under my pillow entered my dreams. That's how I had the idea of actively testing the effect on my dreams of objects that belonged to other people. To do this, I asked my friends to bring me some objects pertaining to their friends without telling me who these friends were. I experienced with these objects, and in ninety-nine percent of the cases, I dreamed of information about the owners of these objects. Of course, if I had dreamed about something private that people would not want to talk about, I did not mention this information. Some psychics can do it in the waking state, and that is called psychometry. Instead, I do it easily and naturally when I sleep with an object next to my head or placed under my pillow. Everyone can do it because our body naturally captures the information of everything around us. At night, this information enters our dreams and reaches our conscious mind. There is no need to be a medium. It is natural for our bodies to capture information about our environment, and it is part of our self-preservation instinct, but many people have never paid attention to this natural phenomenon. The objects belonging to other persons, especially those that have been worn on the skin, are filled with the atmosphere, the energy, the thoughts, the information of their owners, and store this information for a while. If a person is used to dreaming and sleeping well, the objects she uses daily are filled with the energy that emerges from these circumstances. This is why they can help other people to tune themselves with good dreaming and quality sleep. Placing under your pillow or on your night table, an object belonging to some people who are good dreamers will stimulate your ability to dream. The only drawback of this method is that often the dreams you will have will be about the person who lent you the object. But the goal of this technique is to restart the dream function that has been blocked in you. In general, the hardest thing is to start remembering the first dream, so it does not matter what you dream about at the beginning. After that restarting, you will see your dream abilities awaken gradually, and you will be able to maintain your dream ability throughout your life. It is not true that old people no longer dream because of their age. They just stop dreaming because their body is "dirty," especially their digestive system. Let them clean their body through fasting and colonic irrigations, and they will recover their dreaming abilities and, of course, improve their memory. I have now finished with the external boosts. If all the solutions proposed so far did not work for you, it means that there are obstacles that you will have to try to eliminate before you can remember your dreams. These obstacles can come from:

- psychological or physical traumas,

- substances that you consume and that prevent the brain from functioning in a normal way,

- substances that influence your hormonal balance,

- a place where you sleep where energies are unfavorable to sleep, dreams, and vitality.

Therefore, it will be necessary to strive to eliminate or minimize these obstacles to be able to reactivate the memory of your dreams.

# CHAPTER 3: Remove the psychological, material and energetic obstacles that prevent you from remembering your dreams

## 1) The physical and energetic obstacles to recalling your dreams that come from the bedroom and the bed

The material conditions in which you sleep can hinder the memory of your dreams. Like living things, our beautiful planet Earth is not only material. It also has an energy dimension. The Earth is crossed by energy networks. It also receives and exchanges energy with its close environment and the other planets of the solar system. From time immemorial, some people have been aware of the existence of these terrestrial energy networks, and they took them into account to build their houses, their temples, or to establish their cities. These terrestrial energy networks are now called Hartman's networks in the West and the dragon's veins in the East. There are various techniques to detect the crossings of the Hartmann network and the energy disturbances that they can cause. Sensitive people and animals are able to sense through their bodies the path of these nets in their waking state. Everybody can do it easily in the dream state.

In the remote past, no house would have been built without checking the energy properties of the intended place of construction. The ancient Romans, for example, let some geese live for a year on the land where they were planning to build. After a year, the animals were killed and their liver attentively observed because they believed it had the property of reproducing the mapping of the subsoil. Poor animals. Instead of killing them, it would have been enough for some people trained in the art of dreaming to go to sleep in these places and collect this information themselves through their dreams and observe the reactions of their body to this environment. From this, it can be seen that ancient Rome had already lost a great part of the older knowledge possessed by the former inhabitants of the Earth. Today, the situation is much worse because, most of the time, we only take into consideration the financial aspects of construction, and we build without taking into account the cosmo-telluric aspects and the energy networks of the site. This is why many modern homes do not favor good sleep and/or dream recall. If you do not sleep well and do not dream well when you are at home, but if instead, you sleep better and remember your dreams when you do not sleep at home, your problems may come from your home or from your bed. If you sleep in a bed placed above a crossing of telluric energies, this may trigger sleep disorders, and you may feel tired even if you sleep long enough, and of course, you may have difficulties remembering your dreams.

Some crossings of energy nets, the presence of underground cavities and watercourses under the house can be harmful to your health and hinder your ability to dream and sleep well. In this case, change the location of your bed and try different ones until you are able to sleep normally. You will end up finding a good place for your bed that will be good for your health. Too bad if the new, more favorable position of the bed is not aesthetic or practical. You will at least have found a solution, and your health matters much more!

If you wish, during the day, when you do not use it, you may put your bed in the more aesthetic initial position. This type of problem related to cosmo-telluric energies can also be exacerbated by your bedding because of the metal spring mattresses, metal bases and metal frames that all disturb the electromagnetic field of the human body. These types of beds are really not recommended. Instead, choose a bed, a mattress, sheets and blankets made of natural, hypoallergenic materials. Avoid everything metallic in the bed frame. The choice of our bedding is important.

We never emphasize it enough; it is obvious that to sleep well, we need a good mattress adapted to our body type and a good pillow that will ensure that the cervical vertebrae are in an optimal position so that the blood and nervous flows to our brain are not hindered. It is not the most expensive and fashionable bedding that is always the best. Know yourself, observe your dreams and your sleep, and you will know what kind of bedding is best for you. Well-suited bedding will put you in optimal conditions to sleep well, recharge better nervously, and remember your dreams. Also, make sure that your room is well ventilated, that it receives light and air during the day and is dark enough at night. Obscurity relaxes the eyes. Place your bed as far as possible from all electrical appliances, as these continue to emit radiation even when they are turned off. The bed should ideally always be positioned as far as possible from electrical outlets, but this is rarely the case in modern homes. If you have any outlets around your bed and do not sleep well, it would be advisable to switch them off for the night directly at the source, i.e. from the electric meter. You will sleep better, and you will better remember your dreams. In your room, avoid facing reflective surfaces like windows and mirrors that are not conducive to good rest and good sleep. If there are any that you cannot remove, cover them for the night. Of course, it is not advisable to sleep with the cell phone on and placed on the night table, or worse, under the pillow because it will disturb your brain. If you need to leave the phone on, move it away from your head as much as possible. Radio alarm clocks, televisions, tablets, and computers should not be in a bedroom at night. If you cannot avoid that, turn them off for the night, unplug them and cover their screens with a cloth.

We have seen that to facilitate dream recall, the brain must remain passive as in a state of meditation and receptive to what is happening in your body, within you, when you wake up. In this respect, using a radio alarm clock to wake up will prevent you from remembering your dreams because a radio alarm clock makes the brain as active as in the waking state as soon as you wake up.

In addition to the material obstacles associated with the bedroom, there are material obstacles associated with the intake of certain substances and of some allopathic drugs.

## 2) Obstacles to the memory of dreams due to stimulants and drugs:

It is well known that tea, coffee, alcohol, and tobacco are unfavorable to sleep and to the memory of dreams. What is often unknown is that drugs such as contraceptives that influence the hormonal balance can also disturb sleep and prevent a good memory of dreams. It is up to you to experiment to find out which of the substances you regularly use are susceptible to preventing you from dreaming. Of course, be aware, you cannot suddenly stop the intake of some drugs without risks, and if you want to break free of them, you should first seek the help of an experienced doctor. For women who take contraceptives, try to stop taking them for a while. You will remember your dreams much better, and you will also be able to observe what happens in the dream state when natural ovulation occurs. You will also notice which of your dreams announce your ovulation and your menstruation. Tranquilizers and antidepressants have the sad result of almost always suppressing the ability to remember some dreams. However, despite these disastrous circumstances, there are fairly resilient people who are able to dream from time to time while on drugs. I am not hostile to allopathic medicines; they can be very useful in cases of emergencies, for extremely old people, or to avoid unnecessary suffering. But it is a pity to take drugs for insomnia or depressions when you are young. Many other possibilities are at your disposal to rebalance your body and your life to recover natural sleep and the balance of your nervous energy. If you take antidepressants, sleeping pills, blood pressure medications, large amounts of alcohol, tobacco, coffee or tea, you will need to detoxify yourself to start dreaming again. All these substances tend to block the ability to recall your dreams.

In the West, we believe that without medication, it is impossible to cure or alleviate certain diseases. In the past, when these drugs did not exist, doctors used other means that had the advantage of not having side effects and of not blocking the dream activity. I'm not saying that you need to exclude all allopathic drugs. They can be useful in some cases, provided they do not make you dependent on them and are only used for short periods. "Medical drug addiction" is not desirable, even with respect to blood pressure problems. In this regard, I would like to point out that many people say goodbye to their blood pressure problems when they clean their body with colonics and fasting. If you are dependent on drugs and you are too old, it is never too late to change this situation and regain the freedom to live normally and, above all, to dream, but do not take this step lightly and alone. You need to consult professionals who will help you detoxify your body.

In the United States, there are associations of doctors who help patients get out of their addiction to allopathic drugs. A few years ago, I had tried in vain to find in France this kind of structure for one of my consultants. She was about forty and had been taking antidepressants for twenty years, that is, since her mother's death. This person had also tried to find such a structure on her own but had found nothing in France. Later, she told me about some clinics in Russia she had heard about on television, in which, thanks to fasting under medical supervision, it is possible to get rid of drugs.

There are also fasting clinics in other countries, including Germany. One must be very motivated to go to a clinic to fast for a very long time. When one becomes aware of the importance of dreaming, one realizes that the worst that can happen to a human being is to live without dreams and without being aware of one's inner life. When he has lost contact with his inner world and has stopped remembering his dreams, a human being has become a mere kind of robot, a prisoner of his physical body jolted by the circumstances of his environment. Fortunately, in 99% of cases and whatever its initial situation, a motivated person will always be able to recover all or part of her dreaming capacities and to develop them. This will allow her to live her true life and rediscover her true personality and her freedom.

I have never been to a fasting clinic, but of course, I have done all sorts of experiments to observe on my own the effect of fasting on dreams and sleep. During these experiments, I understood why so many religions prescribed fasting and why in the ancient temples of Aesculapius, the pilgrims had to fast. Fasting has a very powerful effect on dreams. When we fast, we sleep much better, and dreams are much clearer and brighter. We remember them much more easily. Why not try it? It's worth it! You may read a book on fasting and experience fasting on your own or join one of the many fasting groups that exist everywhere in the world and that are easily found on the Internet.

3) Psychological blocks to the memory of dreams

**a) Emotional traumas**

Some childhood traumas, such as fear of monsters, reaction to a violent and scary movie, to quarrels and violence in the family, may have caused a disconnection between the "conscious mind" and the "subconscious minds" of a child and settled in the psyche the fear of dreaming.

Adults who dreamed normally as children can also stop dreaming after living a traumatic event in adult life. They usually do not remember any dream even when they sleep enough and in the best possible conditions. When the dreaming abilities are blocked by trauma, the trauma must first be cleared. It may respond very well to acupuncture, especially when applied to a part of your body where the trauma has blocked your energy. You may also use doctor Bach's homeopathic remedy called the rescue remedy. Putting a few drops of this product into some water and ingesting it, incredibly, will help bring to the surface some deeply buried emotions and help you heal your trauma. For a more important trauma that has resisted the previous remedies, you will need the help of qualified professionals.

Through observation of the dream process, it can be noticed that some traumas are transgenerational, which is to say that some traumas can pass from one generation to another. For example, in her book, a psychologist tells the story of a disturbed child who was designing gas masks, which he had never seen before. After some research, it was found that her grandfather had died during the war in the trenches where he had worn the kind of mask that the child had drawn.

A current transgenerational psychology exists that helps patients free themselves from disturbing family memories that often lead to recurring nightmares or block dream recall. If you are interested in the subject, I suggest you read Anne Ancelin Schützenberger's book, which gives many interesting examples of these types of traumas: *The Ancestor Syndrome: Transgenerational Psychotherapy and the Hidden Links in the Family Tree*.

## b) Other blocks to the recall of dreams due to our behaviors

People who lie, who are negative, parasites, disrespectful of themselves of others, their environment, and their body, usually do not show a great interest in dreaming. Of course, as dreams and reality are interconnected, their dreams are not pleasant at all, and they prefer not to remember them. To have pleasant, beautiful, good, bright dreams, one must put oneself in the right psychological conditions. In ancient Egypt, for example, it was known that lying was detrimental to the circulation of energy in the body and in human society. The ancient Egyptians said that lying was the abomination of the gods. At the same time, they did not judge liars and did not try to make them feel guilty or expiate their sins. They did not have our Judeo-Christian mentality. They were pragmatic, and for them, the notion of sin and the sense of guilt associated with it did not seem of any use. Instead, they believed that the best was to become aware of how detrimental some attitudes are to want to abandon them. The ancient Egyptians believed it was always possible to change a wrong attitude, improve oneself and conform to the laws of life. It is interesting to find that Dr. William H. Bates, the American ophthalmologist of whom I have already spoken before, had observed that the sight of human beings instantly decreases when they lie, a phenomenon that he noticed by observing the eyes of his patients with a retinoscope. I quote him: "Even more revealing, a person can have a good sight when he tells the truth, but if she says something wrong, even without the intent to deceive, or even if she imagines a wrong thing, then an eye malfunction occurs or an error of refraction: Experience shows that man is made in such a way that it is impossible for him to say or imagine something wrong without a particular involuntary effort, which is a tension" (Dr. William H. Bates, *A perfect view without glasses, without treatment or intervention*).

# **CONCLUSION**

We have reached the end of this book, which presented you with an array of solutions to resume remembering your dreams. I hope that, thanks to this information, many of you will be able to start dreaming normally and will enjoy a "dream life" and better communication with the inner self that ensues!

When you have recovered your ability to recall your dreams, please go on!

Developing yourself in the "art of dreaming" will change your life. It will render it magical.

In my books listed below, you will find valuable information to help you grow safely and efficiently in the "art of dreaming."

It is truly in my heart to make people dream again, and I am so "contagious" that it often happens that after attending one of my lectures, reading my books, or watching my YouTube videos, people spontaneously resume remembering their dreams after a long time without dreaming. I am so happy to hear about them!

Best wishes to you and have a waking life enhanced by many, many wonderful dreams!

Anna Mancini

# OTHER BOOKS IN ENGLISH BY ANNA MANCINI (www.amancini.com)

They are published by Buenos Books America, and available on Amazon and www.buenosbooks.us

-The Meaning of Dreams

-Your Dreams Can Save Your Life: How and Why Yours Dreams Warn You of Every Danger: Tidal Waves, Tornadoes, Storms, Landslides, Plane Crashes, Assaults, Attacks, Burglaries

- Your Dreams Can Save Your Health: Signs of Infectious Diseases in Dreams, Dreaming the Right Remedies, Accurate Diagnosis, and Early Detection of Diseases

-Depression and How your Dreams can Help you avoid it

-The Clairvoyance of Dreams: What clairvoyance is and how you can simply use your dreams to achieve it

-Tricks to Remember your Dreams

-Tricks to Sleep Better

-Maat revealed, philosophy of justice in ancient Egypt

-How to unlock the secrets, enigmas and mysteries of Ancient Egypt and other old civilizations

-Internet Justice, philosophy of law for the virtual world

-Copyright law is obsolete

-International patent law is obsolete

-Scientific creativity

- Ancient roman solutions to modern legal issues, the example of patent law

# ABOUT ANNA MANCINI

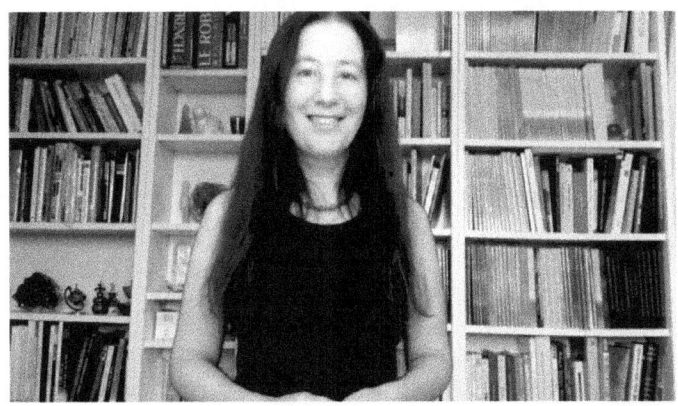

www.amancini.com

Inspired by her family culture, Anna Mancini has been interested in dreams from a young age.

Later, while she was writing her PhD thesis on patent law, a great dream changed her life. This special and very clear dream gave her the solution to a mystery of ancient Roman law that many researchers all over the world had not managed to solve.

For many years she has observed dreams and also dreamers, and has done experiments in order to understand what influence their environment and lifestyle have on the content of their dreams. For her research, she has also made use of old unknown teachings on the human psyche that have survived through the remains of old legal systems.

Thanks to this original method of working on dreams and with the help of her own dreams that have guided her throughout her research, she has been able to:

- develop an innovative and efficient method for the interpretation of oneiric language;

- develop a technique that allows us to ask our subconscious questions and receive answers, whatever the subject area;

- understand which conditions are favorable and unfavorable for creative dreams;

- and discover many other things that make our waking life easier and increase the vitality of dreamers.

She created the research organization 'Innovative You' in 1995, based in Paris, within which she has been able with others to experiment with the techniques for working on dreams that she has developed after long personal research.

She runs workshops, gives lectures and coaches people so that they too can use their dreams to improve all aspects of their lives and also become more creative. She teaches these oneiric creativity techniques in France and abroad, in particular in the research and innovation departments of companies.

# CONTENTS

INTRODUCTION ........................................................ 3

**CHAPTER 1: The ABCs to remembering your dreams** .................................................................... 7

1) It is important to sleep long enough to be able to remember your dreams well. ........................... 8

2) At what time do you have your dinner? What do you usually eat for dinner? And how long after your dinner do you go to sleep? ........................... 14

3) How do you generally wake up? ..................... 17

**CHAPTER 2: Boosts to better remember your dreams** ................................................................. 23

1) Boost to grasp some dreams, images or snippets of your dreams .................................................... 23

2) Material boosts to remember your dreams: ..... 34

3) External dream recall boosters ........................ 41

**CHAPTER 3: Remove the psychological, material and energetic obstacles that prevent you from remembering your dreams** ................................ 53

1) The physical and energetic obstacles to recalling your dreams that come from the bedroom and the bed ....................................................................... 53

2) Obstacles to the memory of dreams due to stimulants and drugs: ............................................ 58

3) Psychological blocks to the memory of dreams 62

CONCLUSION ......................................................... 67

**OTHER BOOKS IN ENGLISH BY ANNA MANCINI (www.amancini.com)** ...................................................... 69

**ABOUT ANNA MANCINI** ................................................... 71

www.ingramcontent.com/pod-product-compliance
Lightning Source LLC
Chambersburg PA
CBHW071313060426
42444CB00034B/2178